LORD YOU ARE MY STRENGTH

From Adversity to Triumph

Orlando Miller
A.K.A.
Landlord

Landlord

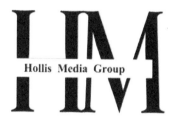

Hollis Media Group
Publisher

Landlord

TABLE OF CONTENTS

ANNOTATIONS

Beloved, let us fearlessly and confidently and boldly draw near to the throne of grace----the throne of God's unmerited favor (to us sinners); that we may receive mercy (for our failures) and find grace to help in good time for every need----appropriate help and well-timed help, coming just when we need it.

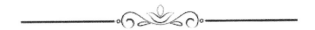

DEDICATION

This book is dedicated to every person struggling with intellectual disabilities and other physical limitations.

Also, to my number one love, my wife and children and my wonderful mother.

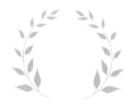

Landlord

Chapter 1

Abandoned
in
The Womb

Here is the beginning of my story. My name is Orlando Miller, also known as Landlord. I was born in the Bahamas. This book is filled with numerous sensitive moments about my early family life and our darkest struggles in the Caribbean: homelessness, being hungry, and often chastised by my stepfather. For the first 10-11 years of my life I grew up thinking the man I called dad was my real father, but he was not... Needless to say, life was busy and messy. My sole purpose for sharing my journey as awkward as it has been is to provide a glimpse of hope, to empower and encourage individuals to never give up. And never allow the adversary to smother your dream because life will get better. Though sometimes it takes a long time, change will come.

Worth reminding . . . We know confession is good for the soul, it cleanses the air and removes dark veils that often keep you emotionally bound and unproductive.

Though the effects are deeply rooted or buried in our subconscious, however, the manifestations can be catastrophic and prevent you from creating and developing meaningful relationships.

For millions who live in *"shame"* when it is never identified or spoken of as such, it is the norm that folks get accustomed to processing. It affects your core: It erodes confidence and self-esteem and diminishes your ultimate outlook on life.

It's akin to a functional addict. You just get up and keep it moving as life is happening. You live in the moment and make snap decisions without factoring that every decision has consequences.

For the most part, you live numb and detached from your emotions and cannot empathize with others who suffer the same fate of misfortune.

Some are wondering about this chapter title, Abandon in the Womb. Well, here is my confession.

My mother, then a young 18-year-old *bright-eyed* Island Girl from Jamaica came to visit the Bahamas with a group of friends for vacation. And as with all young people, she was full of ideas and aspirations to enjoy life. Considering her turbulent home environment back in Jamaica the Bahamas was truly a paradise even if it was going to be short-lived. Being away from her family back home was a welcome change she needed.

My mother was the eldest of her siblings and being the oldest she had a lot of responsibilities to help with house chores and so on. Many times, as a young girl and into her early teens she had to be the babysitter. She was smothered with obligations. Life was difficult. Mom's home setting was consistently saturated with broken communication between her and her mom, and siblings. There were always arguments and disagreements. They argued with ease. She often said how it was unbearable to be around them at times and could not wait to leave.

Surprisingly, while on vacation she met a man who was from Haiti; they hit it off and fell in love.

Eventually, they got married, and that union blessed them with the presence of *three* beautiful children. I wasn't one of them.

After some time passed, the deeply buried issues with my mom began to become more prevalent, she was bipolar. And she did not handle change very well.

Unfortunately, she did not have a great relationship with her family. She and her mother, my biological grandmother did not get along well.

She, too, struggled with bipolar syndrome. **Bipolarism** runs in our family and there was minimum support at best. Back then, Black people did not readily embrace seeing a therapist to address psychological or emotional issues. It was taboo. So, many did not seek out medical treatment and found alternative ways to cope. Drinking was one of them.

Although, if you were deeply religious you prayed about everything . . .You anointed yourself with oil, fasted, read Scriptures but you did not seek a doctor because many believed that constituted you did not have faith. Whew!

As I got older, I realized the tremendous struggle my mother encountered growing up. Her predicament to keep herself moving forward and dealing with a parent who also suffered from the same mental illness was a deal-breaker.

I mean, how do you develop a positive outlook when you are always cast down? When no one has a plan to enrich your spirit to be your ultimate best?

As well as every person of color knows the stigma of being mentally unstable in Black culture is frowned upon. My mom's condition was *UNMENTIONABLE.* It was a closet secret.

In the Black culture, we hid our sick . . . years ago family members and caregivers made sure those who were mentally *impaired* did not mingle socially on the same level. So, Mom detached herself from her family... she did not call as much or communicate as often, the strain in communicating back home forced her to put some distance between them. Though she loved her mother, my grandmother very much they just did not get along.

It took many years for me to understand the social impact mental illness plays. How families have been ripped apart and one's dreams are derailed or die when there is no support system or treatment in place.

In addition, the toll demonic forces have upon life when you are not spiritually covered. No one makes it in life without God's help. Even if you are a sinner, you are living under God's grace and mercy as to why you have not been consumed.

So, if you think it's you alone making the moves and calling the shots, take another look. We control nothing. We are participants given *allowances* to engage life with individual rights to choose to accept His goodness or ignore... But any good thing we enjoy in this life comes from above.

As time progressed my mother and then stepfather was a little financially overwhelmed with raising three children. My stepfather was an auto body worker and my mother did not work. He was the only breadwinner in the family.

Mom was in her early twenties at the time and wanted to go back to Jamaica to visit her family. I surmise this was her way of getting some downtime and giving my stepfather a little space as well.

However, while visiting back home in Jamaica she met a young 17-year-old boy. He was tall and handsome. My mom really liked the young man and he was fond of her as well, but he lied to her about his age. He told her he was 20; his height allowed him to pass for being older.

Well, as you would imagine the unthinkable happened; she had an affair with the 17-year-old and a few months later discovered she was pregnant. What a mess!

Her *predicament* was dire: she was married, already had 3 children back in Nassau and this kid has nothing to offer. She could lose everything. I imagined the thought of having to return to live with her mom in Jamaica must have also scared her beyond belief.

My mother realizing the terrible situation she had landed herself in concocted a plan to get rid of me.

This is the abandonment in the womb. She wrote me off and out of her life. But as we know very well, God had another plan.

I think she believed because my biological father was only 17 that he would not be too hard to convince to support her having an abortion. She was wrong.

She went to the hospital to discuss having a procedure and called my father to bring her some money. After telling him why she needed the money he vehemently refused. He told her "No way would I help you kill my first child". And since she was unemployed and without any financial means to pay, she ended up carrying the pregnancy to term.

Of course, she lamented about how difficult this would be for them and she could not return to Nassau pregnant being a married woman. Yet, he refused.

Eventually, mom returned home to Nassau and intertwined the pregnancy into her scheme to conceal the affair and put me off on my stepfather. Though I grew up many years believing he was my biological father. We had a great relationship and I know he loved me as best as he could. There are many fond memories.

As I grew older many neighbors and family members became suspicious and talk began to spread about me not having much resemblance to my dad or siblings.

The Dichotomy . . .

It was a dilemma because my siblings were darker and my complexion was fairer so people gossiped. And I'm certain my stepfather had to eventually acknowledge the probability of their speculations.

I guess I was around 5 years old when my mother decided to make another visit back to Jamaica and she brought me with her. On this trip, I met my biological dad. Wait, it gets deeper. Don't release the balloons or cut the cake yet. There were *anomalies*.

It would be an understatement if I said the trip was uneventful. There were several surprises, things my little mind could not process. While visiting Jamaica I lived with my biological father (*though I had no idea he was my father*) and his Fiancée.

I have no idea how my mother pulled this off but I remained in Jamaica for a little while and was enrolled in first grade. I imagined I was there for about 1 year.

Well, at the age of 5 it felt weird to me when the gentleman I now lived with began introducing me as his son. He took me around several of his friends and acquaintances and would say to them, "I want you to meet my son." And I would say to him, *"You are not my dad. My father is back home in Nassau."* I could only work with the limited knowledge I had...

Though the feelings I had were perplexing because I thought why this man is lying about me being his son. I was too young to organize my thoughts to articulate just how unpleasant I felt about him pretending to be my dad.

After some time, my mother took us back to Nassau. I felt a sense of belonging through the tension in our home that was thick enough to slice with a dull butter knife. Whatever was going on between my dad (stepfather) and she was reaching a boiling point. With 4 mouths to feed, keeping a roof over our heads, clothed, and a host of other things they were dealing with was unraveling their marriage. The limited structure they were enjoying was slipping away.

I'm not sure what had taken place between my parents and what was discussed in many of their conversations about mom's last trip to Jamaica, and about me, but something had to happen.

A few years passed, and I remember being around 11 years old when my mother one day said to me she needed to share something. Well, her tone was different, and I thought to myself what could possibly be wrong now.

Thoughts were racing in mind since we had a very unstable lifestyle. I knew the sky would fall just didn't know when. I tried to prepare myself. Since we moved a lot because my parents could barely afford to be consistent with rent that was one thought that came to mind. So, I braced myself for what was about to be said. My heart started beating a little faster as she slowly summoned the courage to tell me what was on her mind.

She pulled me aside and said, "I want you to know the man you stayed with in Jamaica is your father." What! How is that possible? I thought. So, she went on to tell me that my stepfather was not my biological dad among other things that I did not care to know.

Having learned of my traumatic beginning being abandoned in the womb where she put in motion a plan to kill me, was still fresh. Yes, I was abandoned from the womb. In her mind, she separated me as a human being to perhaps just tissue without a soul, or purpose in the world.

Why was I not valuable enough? Why would a married woman seek love in a younger man? Too many queries and all above my comprehension at that stage.

In a way I thought why would she mess things up like this, though life with my stepfather wasn't easy but how would this young man now in his twenties provide any better for her, and her 4 children?

In the mind of every little boy, no one compares to his Mama. She is the Queen; strategic problem solver, the SAGE, the wonderful culinary chef (*even if the food is not that great, but hey, we learn to deal . . . you're your mom*).

In addition, one's mom represents the essence of all things sweet. The one who kisses the boo-boos, teaches you how to wipe your runny nose and always reminds you to brush your teeth after every meal. To take care of what is most important.

Your Mama is supposed to be the *molder-in-chief* who prepares your spirit to be strong; to face every crisis and helps you to recognize open opportunities and go after them with all your passion. She is indelibly the prize of God's creation.

To me, this is what I wish could be said of my experience as a child growing up in the Bahamas. My family was of modest means; we had to make do as did all families in similar stations but our family nucleus had several layers of *daunting* complexity.

Our family dynamic included a tethered secret that hung around our necks like a cylinder block obstructing the sunshine of childhood bliss. We lacked the experience of being carefree, and dreamy. That which was supposed to be the norm was nonexistent for us; children should grow up in households where mom and dad held everything down, including being **blockers** to keep them from being over-exposed to constructs and conversations way upon their level of maturity.

In my day, adults had no problem reminding you when to stay out of grown folks' business. NONE. They protected, as much as they provided.

DARK SECRETS . . .

My mother got married young, she was a typical *Island Girl* full of ambition and dreamed of a better life. To have a family, to be in love, and to see the world. At least this is my narrative.

As children when you are in broken environments you have a way of juxtaposing theories to fit your imagination to deal with pain and disappointment. In actuality, you find an amazing way to build up pain blockers emotionally and psychologically just to function day-to-day.

Nevertheless, due to circumstances beyond my family's control, that is, having a parent with an intellectual disability, by the way, the term *"intellectual disability"* is a genuinely nice posh term nowadays. 20 years ago, the unfavorable term was retarded, crazy, mental, and often slung about in idle gossip or when kids made fun of someone.

As a result of my mom struggling with mental illness what I experienced was unbelievable heartache and shame. Imagine awakening every day in constant fear of what might happen or be said about your mom that is going to piss you off. For me, this was a *primary* feeling, parallel to having my blanket like Linus in *Charlie Brown*. Everywhere I went, the pain and frustration followed. There was no separation because I didn't have the power to change my family dynamics, which was the source of my shame.

Everywhere I went, the blanket, the shame, fear, and loneliness were attached. As well as the silent pain from stifled conversations I entertained in my head but with no one to listen. I became my own therapist, which is never a good thing to diagnosis your health. Mind you, at this stage I am a child growing faster than I care to, but the trajectory of my life is not in my control. I had to play the hand life dealt...

Now as an adult, a father, and a spiritual leader, it is so difficult for me to look at the suffering of children the same way. When I catch a glimpse of blank stares, eyes with no glimmer or shine, I immediately wonder is this a child crying out for love, support, or an opportunity to belong? To be included in something bigger in life and nurturing?

I ask of myself, are they too, encapsulated into a dark abyss of misunderstanding with nowhere to hide, or to find comfort or encouragement to just keep believing and never stop hoping for change?

I was surrounded by many who could have stepped up and intervened to make some days, not every day, but some of those darkest moments in my childhood a little bit easier, kinder. And a few did.

I can remember one of my friends whose family had a banana farm, he fed me many, many times and made sure I was straight. I am most grateful for his compassion. Our exchanges growing up made a *permanent* impression upon me.

Then there were those antagonistic folks; some adults and many of my peers that would hurl all kinds of insults. They were cruel, and they said cruel things simply because we were poor. It is this kind of experience that causes a child to grow up bitter and hardened. It is emotionally abusive and leaves invisible scars on your mind. Cruelty can snuff out your voice. It makes your soul quiet... You lose footing and live like a Neanderthal; a drifter without purpose.

I can honestly say I was hollow and didn't understand it. How could I, I was just a child. This is what happens when society looks the other way; when we say nothing, do nothing, and shrug off the visual struggles of others before us as just an ordinary moment.

When other kids spoke so well of their mom, I struggled to keep my mom from ever being a part of anyone's conversation. I needed to protect her, but how? Children who learned of my mom's battle with mental illness obviously heard the whispers, and gossip from their moms and grandmothers sitting at the dinner table, or from other kids repeating talks from their home or at the playground.

So as one could imagine my playtime with other kids also meant I had to fight off being bullied, teased, and taunted about my mother's condition. It was another burden and obstruction to my personal growth, the moments when I should have been free, safe, and optimistic in life, many of those days were filled with fear of the unknown.

Do you know what it feels like when someone calls your mom, your queen, retarded, stupid, and crazy? You know all the wonderful adjectives kids whimsically think of at a split second. Those interactions made me cringe and robbed me of my worthiness.

At the sound of each taunt, every foul negative comment made against my dear mother it felt like my heart had been ripped into a thousand pieces. How does a boy handle the nastiness spoken against the one person he *worships* but has no defense for?

I wrestled with my emotions. I used to cry so much, and question God why did you send me through this family?

What would be in the mind of God to assign this fate to me; was this some type of judgment or mistaken identity? I often wondered why so much hurt befell my family.

Growing up was immensely difficult with mom dealing with her instability and my father was not present. This was a plank of death, many times it felt like I would not make it. With all the negativity surrounding me at home, in the neighborhood, at school, there was no escape from this madness that was slowly eroding any confidence and self-esteem I tried to muster.

Each time I built myself up, there were instances that blew on that foundation causing me to start over, and over, and over. Life seemed cruel, God felt distant, and as much as I lamented within even, he, appeared unconcerned about a little black hunger boy. A child who so much just wanted to have stability and be the apple of his mother's eye, instead of having to fight every day just to breathe.

In my then limited ability to comprehend life compared the differences in family paradigms. Instinctively, I knew there were different types of family structures, some seem to have everything.

My perspective about my family was not so rewarding. I saw brokenness and did not know what it was, but I felt it. Lived it. And cried every night to get away from the pain that was sucking the life out of me.

When you are born into brokenness, live in brokenness, and folks around you are selectively oblivious to first pause to see if you are okay, and secondly when it is in their power to help, to do so, but don't. Now what? Because life is a continuum and nothing is stopping just because you got problems, you have to learn on your feet, quickly or get squashed in the process.

Chapter 2

Life in the Grove

I grew up near *Wulf Road* and Wrights Lane. It was located in the Grove (the Ghetto), this was not an easy area to raise a family. Besides being in abject poverty, I had a mother who frequently came unhinged. I had 2 brothers and 3 sisters. We spent many years eating little of nothing. We did not have lavish dinners like other families or take vacations from the island. We were at the bottom economically.

Our holidays were vastly different; we never had an abundance of things (food, toys, clothes etc.,) to enjoy like other families. I can remember many Christmas mornings there was nothing under the tree. Heck, we did not even have a tree.

There were several Thanksgivings without a turkey and the traditional foods families would normally share. And other families looked down upon others. The kids were brutal...

I remember one Christmas we did not have any food to eat. The only food we had in the cupboard was rice. My stepfather went to the store and bought some sweet cream, and rice. He mixed them together, it was the first time we ate porridge.

What I now know and understand is everyone hits a wall. No matter how *deep* you perceive your walk to be, this journey in life consists of zigzags, pitfalls, ebbs and highs.

There are moments when you feel abandoned, unloved, live seemingly unprotected and without any solid plan for the future. But know this is just a moment . . . Nothing, and hear me clearly, NOTHING can overturn the plan of God for your life, except if you choose not to possess it. And yes, you will have to fight by faith.

My family's struggle was austere, we were always moving. We were like *Caribbean Gypsies.* Though the rent in one apartment was only *$30* dollars a week my parents could barely meet the obligation.

One time the landlord was so tired of my family being behind in the rent that he took off the front and back doors exposing us to the elements. The structure was linear, you could see straight through from the front to the back of the house.

This was as embarrassing as the neighbors and my peers watched our life spiral downward. As a kid this was traumatic.

The Landlord felt that he would make life as miserable as possible for my family to force us to leave. Keep in mind, my family had nowhere else to go. So, we hung curtains to keep people from looking in, and at night we had to sleep right by the doors to prevent burglars from coming in to steal. Though we experienced many break-ins and people eventually stole what little we possessed, we were always starting over to some degree. There was never any consistent longevity or duration in stability. Our lifestyle was fluid. Any day, at any time, it could be feast or famine.

We barely had electricity in the house because my parents could not afford to pay so we lived for periods by candles and Kerosene lanterns. This also meant we could never have any perishable food in the refrigerator to store.

Without question this was immensely distressing. We were teased a lot. And my mom being bipolar would often explode and cuss out the neighbors and say whatever came to mind. The adage: *what comes up comes out.* She was free flowing that way.

My siblings and I would be so humiliated and often tried to distance ourselves from her so no one would think she was our mother.

I'll never forget when she came to my school wearing 3 different shades of lip stick all over her face, I was mortified. My siblings and I hid. We did not acknowledge her presence; it was too *exasperating.* Seemingly she could not process that because of her and the way we lived I had such low self-esteem.

Some kids commit suicide over this kind of upbringing, but I know it was only God's grace that kept me moving forward because at that time I had no one, and nothing to comfort me the way I really desired.

I literally hated my life and the way I was forced to accept certain things. It robbed me of my confidence. And having a mom with mental issues people always teased me about her being retarded and crazy and all sorts of negative talk.

I asked God time-after-time, WHY? Why am I in this family ... Why couldn't you give me another family! And to make matters worse for us kids, my mom was from Jamaica and my stepfather was Haitian so they were both considered foreigners. It was rough. The Bahamians people did not take too kindly to foreigners that could not pull their own weight.

People used to tell them to get out of their country, that they were not welcome in the Bahamas. Of course, mom, being bipolar she would cuss everyone out. It made matters worse for us.

There were many times I wished I could just fall asleep and not wake up. This had to be the worse and longest nightmare of my life, and I was tired of living it. I pleaded with God to do something for me, don't leave me in this hell hole.

Now, when I hear stories of people's struggle so many are mild compared to what we had to endure. We grew up without a lot of basic necessities... I remember we had to all share the same toothbrush. C'mon man. Now that's a struggle.

There are so many thoughts surrounding having to put a used toothbrush in my mouth . . . I try to block thoughts of that experience as much as possible. Certainly, it's not something I would ever do again, no matter.

This was no way for a child to live but it was our reality for a long time. Also, it was years before I had a bathing towel. Something as *rudimentary* as a bath towel to wash myself my parents couldn't even afford.

Can you imagine in order to clean up I would use my torn underwear to wash myself, and then put my wet underwear back on?

Some of my friends would ask, "Landlord, why are your pants always wet?" I could not tell them it was because I bathed with my underwear. I had to do what I had to do.

Even as I am writing to retell what I passed through my eyes constantly well up. I am humbled and grateful to God for His hand being upon my life (*though this awareness was foreign to me).*

As I reflect on this massive dark hole in my life, I can imagine the anguish others are yet processing and about to take a dark turn for the worse. This is what fueled my desire to get this book into the universal space that would serve as a testament of God's redeeming power. To prove that God's plan always come to the light for He cannot alter the words spoken out of His mouth.

Therefore, we must learn in every season to summon faith, and courage to press beyond the present. No matter what, let us remember when the enemy comes in like a flood the Lord will raise a standard against Him! The devil just doesn't want you to realize how loved you are so he assaults your mind. Remember, the adversary knows Scripture too. He knows the word says, "As a man thinketh so is He".

When you lack this insight, fear is always present with you. There is constant bombardment of warring thoughts you will have to organize, eliminate, and dominate to live constructively because the enemy comes to steal the center of your peace.

As a result of all the adversity happening so rapidly in my life, I questioned God so much. I repeatedly asked why He couldn't have given me a different family... WHY not me? Why couldn't I have good fortune and enough to eat? Nice clothes, a bike to ride to school etc.

The wounds were deep from the embarrassing encounters. Every episode layered on more traumatic thoughts that robbed everything good from my soul.

We were so poor; I had to attend school wearing old clothes; busted pants, busted shoes and sometimes had NO lunch. It was bad. Learning was a struggle because my mind was constantly thinking about what in the world I am going to eat today.

Psychosocial Dynamics in Question

When I was in Junior high, I remember needing a school bag so I wouldn't have to walk to and from school carrying heavy books. Most all of my classmates had school bags. I was the odd one out among my peers and it created a lot of peer pressure.

I repeatedly pleaded with my stepfather to buy me a school bag. Well, what I got from him instead was a briefcase. Not a new one, one of his old ones lying around.

It didn't make any sense ... I did not understand why in the world he gave me a briefcase.

I was teased mercilessly. Kids would come to me and say, "Landlord, why you carrying that briefcase like a businessman, where's your book bag?"

There was already enough preexisting drama to last a lifetime, I didn't need anything else added to my plate of misery and misfortune. The store shelves in those departments were adequately stocked.

In addition to all the other layered adversity and *nightmarish* experiences I lived through, I remember needing shoes for school. My parents bought me a cheap pair of black shoes to wear. They were not the best, but it beats having to walk to school in my bare feet, which I did at times.

When I was home, I walked mostly bare feet so that I would not damage my school shoes. I didn't have a second pair, and the other reason was money was scarce. I knew I had to do my best to take care of my shoes or it could possibly be a long time before getting another replacement pair.

So, I carried super glue with me all the time just in case something fell apart, I would just glue it back on.

Also, my shirts had buttons with so many different colored threads holding them together and boy the kids had a field day with that... it was tough.

The kids that had nicer things were notorious for being cruel. Their precision was impeccable and I often wondered if they gathered for a preamble before school to decide who would say what. They were so proficient in mocking me and my siblings. This would go on before school, during school, after school, and on the weekend.

There was a pronounced absence of concern; they didn't seem to care how badly the teasing made me feel. My misfortune kept them amused. However, I kept fighting in my mind and telling myself "*one day*" this will change.

As one could imagine this type of hostility weighs on you and robs you from the core of your being. It always amazed me that most of them seemed to lack any compassion. But I guess why they would because our economic situation was not their problem. Nevertheless, you would think there would be an ounce of humanity extended. That's always FREE! Just takes a little effort and a conscience.

Attending school was horrible. There was one time when my mother came to the school with 3 different shades of lipstick. My heart almost stopped. Out of all the mockery we kids had to endure she compounded the misery with this side show.

I cannot over emphasize how depressing life was . . . I did not know it then but I was *chronically* depressed. I welcomed any thoughts of escapism that reflected hope, no matter what. I felt anything a little grade above this crazy whirlwind would do me simply fine.

Later on, that desperation to escape got me mixed up with the wrong crowd doing unthinkable acts of cruelty and other illegal activity. In my limited capacity to see clearly, I felt accepted.

Though I knew those boys were not the right people to congregate with but because it appeared they were for me, it was for the wrong reasons. We did a lot of bad things.

The brotherhood was not good. We robbed people and committed other dastardly acts that I am too ashamed to mention in detail. And this is what happens when you lose sight of the big picture or when there is NO compass to guide you morally.

In addition, this is why so many of our abandoned children from broken families are prime candidates for recruitment.

I saw many of my friends/associates murdered. Some went to jail. There was always something catastrophic going on in the ghetto.

I remember when by brother went to jail and him telling me, "Landlord, stay away from that place. This is not where you want to come. Being incarcerated will take more from you than you are willing to give... Your dignity, and hope are on the line. There is nothing good there man. Do something else with your life". I would always tell him I had no plans to go to jail.

A part of me knew he was right, but the other side of the coin reflected a means to an end. I'm not proud to say this, "I robbed people to meet material needs." I tried to fight my conscience. I knew better. But I was also desperate.

I was tired of being hungry all the time and wearing tattered clothes, and old cheap shoes. I wanted to experience something good in my life like other children my age.

I wanted to live in house with a functional bathroom. Our bathroom was always saturated with water, the room leaked. It was a mess.

And as I mentioned earlier, we barely had electricity on a consistent basis so there was never any television shows we were able to enjoy growing up. We might well as have lived in a remote desert since most our lifestyle was primitive. And having NO lights it's kind of hard to entertain yourself in the dark.

Notwithstanding, I can remember being around 3 or 4 and I loved to sing. When I sang it took my mind somewhere else and eased my anxiety. Our home environment was not the most nurturing.

There were equally as many if not more demerits as there were fond times.

Sometimes we just wanted to play outside well, my stepfather did not like us being outside much just in case we had an altercation with the neighbors. Most of them did not like us because they didn't approve of my mother's behavior. We were seen as the bad kids with a crazy mother.

Of course, mom didn't make the situations any easier when she went on her cussing rampages. There were many close calls of a fight breaking out between the adults because of threats and other foolish talk.

Those actions reflected upon us negatively in the community and my parents mostly stayed to themselves as a result.

Chapter 3

Thing Parents Should Recognize

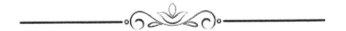

In this chapter I want to share some strategic insight with parents to help you identify the disconnect that happens within your child.

Many times, parents who are themselves challenged with emotional issues and other unaddressed psychological dynamics are prone to overlook the void within their child's life. Some ascertain that their children are wanting too much from them, or that they need to learn how to cope and survive.

One of the biggest misnomers in parenting is when parents make comparative assessments. How they lived vs, how their children are living. Some judge the ability of their children to cope based on how they had to manage and navigate life.

This process can be ruthless and inflict unnecessary pain upon a child's psyche if they are left to interpret life lessons by themselves. We have to help cultivate *Critical Thinking* skills; they are not automatic. A child's environment is primarily connected to his/her world view. When you disavow the impact on children's development being in a predominately negative environment the consequences are going to be grave. There will be manifestations of psychological conflicts within them.

If a child doesn't feel safe, or loved, they will act out just to garner attention. It has never been okay to say, "Oh, they'll get over it or grow out of it." Emotional scars can damage you for a lifetime.

It is a travesty that should never be but unfortunately many children are born into families that poses imminent threats to their life.

As a parent, one of your greatest responsibilities is to ensure your child is safe, nurtured and instructed. When you disconnect emotionally your children feel it. Your primary interaction should not be just to be an Authoritarian presence, but a guide. An investor in their hopes and dreams.

When children feel overlooked depression sets in. They become lethargic, and there will be disruptions in the house, school, and the community.

Understanding now more through my studies I can see the triggers in my mom's life. Just having children is a mental anguish as a result of sleep deprivation and extra pressures in the home.

I know if my stepfather were able to get her treatment some of the misfortune that landed in her way would have glossed over or didn't happen at all. But there wasn't any enlightenment in this area or money to seek it out.

As result, I had to learn to take care of myself. I can remember working at 11 years old.

I can now see the footprint of God in the most distressful times of my life. When I was homeless, which was many, many times. He made provision.

It was always a mystery to me why we could not have a stable home for any length of time.

Unfortunately, there are several misguiding factors when parents with a rough up bringing make comparative assessments with their children. No two people are alike. No one will match your footprint exactly, not even your child. Though there will be similarities but understand your children are given a trajectory by God... "I know the plans I have for you saith the Lord." This God made declaration is the authoritative guide for every person.

Some parents make comparative assessments with their children based on what they experienced and survived as if there were guarantees. Parents shouldn't be comfortable omitting to ensure your home environment is the safest space for your child.

Unproductive environments will always stunt emotional and psychological development. Many childhood traumas, particularly those that are interpersonal (*emotional abuse: EA, emotional neglect: EN, physical abuse: PA, physical neglect: PN, and/or sexual abuse: SA in childhood and/or adulthood*) intentional, and chronic are associated with greater rates of PTSD, PTSS, depression and anxiety, antisocial behaviors and greater risk for alcohol and substance use disorders.

The brief above listing is enough to derail any educated person let alone an unprotected mind of a child.

If you are a parent prone to dismiss emotional duress, the cost of corrective measures can take everything from you, including the life of your child. So don't ignore the warning signs.

Understandably parenting is a monumental task, at times it's overwhelming. So, we don't have to downplay the energy it takes to create a happy home, it requires everything.

No matter if you are religious, spiritually, enlightened, or whatever other label you wear life will present some difficulties that you will have to pray about. The worse thing we do as humans is isolate ourselves. This is the devil's playground. You have to get connected.

I realize my parents isolated themselves to keep from being in fights and arguments with a few of the neighbors. But cutting yourself off from having positive encounters with others is detrimental.

We need positive input in our lives. People help people grow, develop, expand, and prosper.

If life is getting too daunting, perhaps seeking professional help will allow you the opportunity to reconstruct your home environment that could lend itself to creating positive exchanges between you and your family. This should not be approached lightly. When in trouble, SCREAM!

I wished my mother were capable of asking for assistance when she needed it most. Certainly, my parents were nomads in a foreign country. They were "*Persona non grata*". UNWELCOMED! As result several adults were equally as nasty to us kids.

When parents who struggled immensely during childhood with negative behavior pass on the injustices of their past onto their offspring, this is the blueprint to a paradigm of generational deterioration and massive dysfunction.

We have to discern what triggers are being released that are harmful to the emotional wellbeing of a child and take the necessary steps to help our children forge a strong identity that serves as a basis for finding future direction in life. It's a blueprint.

It is imperative to create environments that are nurturing, spiritual and lends itself to exploration pertaining myriad of subjects. The more structured exposure a child has, the broader their awareness will be of life.

Minimalize the Aint's

Depressive thoughts manifests in various ways: feelings, behavior, and physiology. There are times when we are not present in life to fully appreciate what is taking place in real-time. If our outlook is predominately steeped in futuristic applications or we are always rehearsing the past, neither is conducive to productivity or success.

Likewise, a child, perhaps your child is experiencing one or both of the above as a result of what is taking place in your life **MOM/DAD**.

No matter how inundated you feel, and maybe it's extremely difficult for you at the moment, and there is no village near to turn to. However, we must be cognizant of the seeds being sown into the life of a child. The tenderness and innocence that are being stolen and replaced with deep emotional scars. For the sake of your lineage, your seed, there has to be course-correction

Methodologies that aren't working and are eroding your family nucleus from the inside out, have to **GO!**

Chapter 4

Gifts, Introduction, and Patience

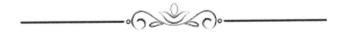

In this chapter I want to segue to say this: You will not always feel the value of your gifts or comprehend the magnitude of the possibilities your gifting could produce. What your gifts contain isn't always readily apparent. However, as you continue to keep exercising faith and explore every option to better yourself, making the word of God your center, the strength needed to climb and leap over any hurdle comes easier. You start to dominate what use to dominate you.

It's amazing how clearer life becomes when you grasp whose you are.

Now, it is necessary to guard your mind and spirit against cynicism when moments in life appear that you aren't progressing or going *NOWHERE.* Practice being open to the whispers of God to speak to your situation through friends, foes, nature. Pay attention.

Many times, your answer comes through unfamiliar things, processes. But your intimacy with God will always lead you to that which is divine, a place of knowing where faith moves mountains, and bring miracles into manifestation in the NOW!

The illusion the devil will consistently paint before you is "YOU don't have what it takes. You came from the wrong stock." Rebuke him.

This is what I know with absolute certainty; your gift will demand the audience (*INTRODUCTION*) it was bestowed to influence if you don't quit or squander opportunities as they are presented.

It means being present (conscious) and curbing the temptation to operate from a futuristic framework (always daydreaming) — this life has to be lived, daily. We were created to be about the business of NOW. We are required to handle "TODAY'S" business while it is today. Fantasizing and prescheduling every moment of the day without allowances of input from God is disastrous. Life is a partnership. Your relationship with God requires *teamwork.* He calls, you follow.

When you begin to operate and flow in your calling there will be an intense struggle to stay focus. The adversary strategically dispatches disruptions to cloud your judgment, to delay your response to a directive given by God in a specific timeframe, and ultimately to get you to uproot your seed.

The devil is *deceitful* opponent, he's been playing this game of deception a very long time. Don't fall for the inpatient trick. The adversary will have you focus on how long you have been waiting, and ain't nothing happening. Or, how much you invested in church work, ministries, paying your tithes and offerings and your land is still barren and pockets empty. Don't fall for the trick. Keep obeying.

Hang in there and allow patience to have "her" perfect work. You have everything to gain and *everything* to lose if you faint. When you move out of sync, out of alignment with God's timing for your life His grace gives you an opportunity to make course corrections quickly, though it is totally up to you to be willing to let go. Other times it could take years to come around again because of the entrapments along the way. Stay in place.

We cannot force the plan; we must align with the plan and the manifestation will come.

Sometimes the disruption and disconnect is as simple as moving ahead of God or procrastinate to make the connection set before you. Either one requires you correct yourself.

In addition, it is paramount to strengthen your focus on the "Principal" thing. First things first. In the life of Christians, it should be Christ.

It should not be a constant practice of saints to skip prayer or reading the word of God. This is the source of your strength. If the devil can get you in a mode of miscommunicating with God, it becomes a primary obstacle to hurdle. You dig deeper in pits that you should have walked out of.

Anytime we decide to get closer to God the enemy bombs your runway. He will fight intensively to keep you from taking off the ground and growing in your faith.

Reaching new dimensions in God takes not only courage but, *stick-to-itiveness.* You have to have a drive to outlast your storm. To consistently see better things happening for yourself. Success is not only NOT automatic, but also a process. And that course will be followed by another process, backed up with several more processes intertwined with zigzags and uncertainty. We have to get use to *CHANGE.* It is inevitable.

However, herein is great consolation: SO, WHAT if you stumbled and lost your footing? We must live sober-minded to fight the good fight of faith and recognize the impending doom the adversary wants you to incorporate by speaking death over your life. To your dreams, your destiny.

We must remember God's word is final. In spite of every pit, every ditch you find yourself stuck in, the promise of God is sure. "I will complete what I started". We have victory even when it appears to have disappeared.

I remember being homeless so many times and sleeping wherever I could find shelter, and certainly there were moments of deep despair.

I could not imagine a loving God being at the helm directing my path because I was met with misfortune, after misfortune. I mean really; what kind of God does this?

Jehovah Jireh? Well, being hungry, homeless and broke didn't register that Jesus had me on the payout that day. I felt overlooked and abandoned.

Chapter 5

Watch what shows up

I cannot emphasis enough the importance of staying in faith; nothing takes the place of having a positive outlook. When you are feeling depleted and out of solutions look at the gifts already in your hand, what you are blessed to do will be the very instrument to liberate your life. To prosper you.

At the age of 5 I knew I loved to sing; singing liberated me by providing an escape from the household drama and other misfortune we were experiencing. When domestic issues escalated, I retreated more to music. It was akin to David in the bible playing the harp to drive away evil spirits when King Saul was tormented. I don't think I would have made many of the positive connections that turned my life around without music. I used to get into so much trouble in school; skipped classes and acted out because of the emotional trauma I was wrapped up with.

Later I started to recognize the calm in my life because of music—it transformed my way of thinking and how I processed my feelings. Actually, I took on a new identity; music brought normalcy.

Having music in my blood made a world of difference and you will discover when you step out in faith using what you have, God honors it. This is why the adversary fights so hard to get folks to lay down their talent, to not honor the gifting or as another way to say this, turn their back to God.

Your transformation is directly tied to allowing the God within to speak, sing, write, act, preach, teach, etc. Use what you have, don't waste time trying to convince the naysayers about anything God has spoken over your life because what they think doesn't matter anyway. Keep your focus.

Chapter 6

God's Way

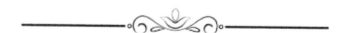

We must conclude that the Word of God is infallible and is the express imagine of God in written form. We can depend upon it, trust it, and share it with those in need and see transformation.

There are some hard places we have to deal with however, God does not change. Your adversity is not your end, but the seed to your triumph.

The success I now enjoy is directly correlated to learning how to hang in there, to consistently push past pain and disappointment and not allow the spirit of hopeless to take root. In addition, I got connected to the right people. My past gave me the development that set me up for my life's journey. I can pinpoint major strengths present in my life directly linked to past difficult moments when it looked like it was over.

When I could have gotten lost in bad behavioral choses God had a person for me. I am a better person, a stronger, wiser man as a result of the path God allowed to unfold for me. I mean before the fame, money or any recognition, the path of hardship and constantly dealing with lack helped me learn how to empathize more quickly with hurting people. One could say the harsh experiences tenderized my heart.

Living in dire situations made me fight with my faith and use the word of God more. I found myself going back to the Bible over and over to grab a hold of a passage or two to help me get through the day. Days eventually turned into months, months into years and soon I was out of that hopeless situation.

Some of you may still be in the midst of what appears to be a hopeless relationship or you're wrestling with family dynamics where there is so much chaos and emotional strife, don't you dare given in. You cannot quit, you must push past the pain and get centered in the Word of God. This is where your safety lies and the answers needed to foster a new beginning. Plus, the added bonus is as your search the Word of God you will find answers.

There are no dilemmas in God. Whatever negative situation is lingering there is a word for it, there is an end on God's schedule to the pain and discomfort --- It's all connected to God's time, purpose and season.

The Lord never saved you to linger, or drag about through life. God called you to move forward, to thrive and live as an example before others in faith and perseverance. What we have to practice doing is shifting attitudes and aiming our energy for a favorable outcome, learn to see the end from the beginning. The bible encourages us to tap into the authority given to us through the word of God; "call those things that be not as though they were".

There is so much we could not include this time but I said to Hollis Media, I know what God has given me and I humbly work within those parameters. As one could imagine there were many edits, rewrites trying to create the right one and message. Certainly, all of this is out of my love for God and his people, you.

So, it is my hope you find your voice and strike out on the journey God called you to and never look back. Never surrender and never live in fear. You got this.

In wrapping this up I want to share one of my deepest desires to serve others, especially talented artists from the Bahamas because so many are given less recognition but they are so talented.

I promised God if he would assist me, to help me establish myself that I would always remember to come back and help those left behind to get the right break. God honored me. Humbly I can say the Lord is using me to bring so many artists from obscurity into the public square on the international stage.

I look at what I do as a ministry; this ministry is launching greatness for the Kingdom of God.

However, here are some of my favorite passages of Scripture that carried me and strengthen my focus.

Proverbs 19:21 - *Many are the plans in a man's heart, but it is the Lord's purpose that shall prevail.*

Proverbs 16:7 -- *When a man's ways please the Lord, he maketh even his enemies to be at peace with him.* ***(King James Translation)***

James 4:10 -- *Humble yourselves in the presence of the Lord, and He will exalt you.*

1 Peter 5:6 - *Therefore humble yourselves under the mighty hand of God, that He may exalt you at the proper time.*

Matthew 23:12 - *Whoever exalts himself shall be humbled; and whoever humbles himself shall be exalted.*

2 Chronicles 7:14 --- *And My people who are called by My name humble themselves and pray and seek My face and turn from their wicked ways, then I will* *hear from heaven, will forgive their sin and will heal their land.*

Proverbs 22:4 -- *The reward of humility and the fear of the Lord are riches, honor and life.*

Romans 8:31 – If God is for us who can be against us.

Psalm 37:23 -- The steps of a good man are ordered by the Lord; and he delighted in his way.

You, are on assignment. God will strengthen you for battles, and strategic assignments to bring deliverance. And He blesses you to be a BLESSING!

When I'm facing things that appear impossible to conquer, I look at the receipts in my life. God bringing me out of abject poverty, giving me a name, and a position to make a difference in the world to influence others to trust him, to dream and to win.

In spite of all that doubted my worth, those who blocked me at different stages of my life, God showed up for me. You are not the labels others placed upon you... See yourself through the eyes of faith and always say what God says about you.

God wants you to know, what folks are doing negatively will not cancel His plan. Your hurt isn't permanent, keep believing. You are going to triumph!

Make the Lord your strength!

GALLERY

Always remember where you started ...

First album release. 1999
"Never forget where you come from".

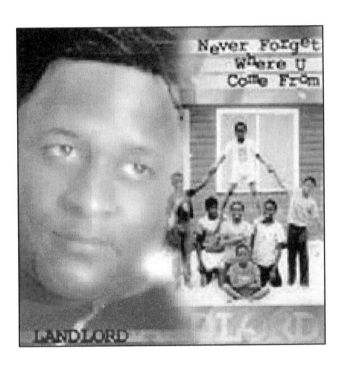

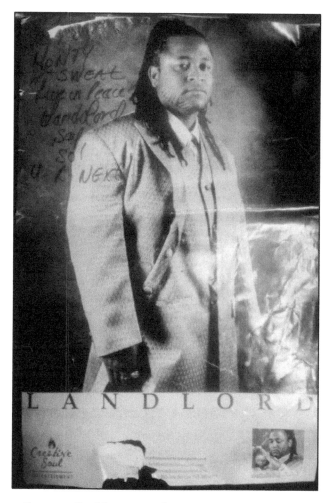

Second album release. 2004
" We need peace".

A man's gift makes room for him and brings him before the GREAT!

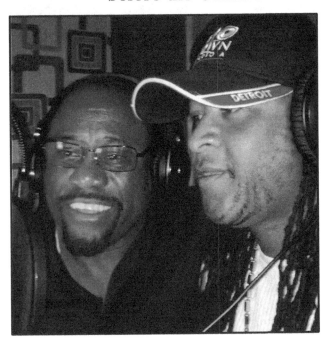

Dr. Myles Munroe & Landlord in studio.
He was featured in the song "All Over the World."

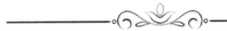

God has done GREAT THINGS!

Stellar Awards 2018 Las Vegas, Nevada

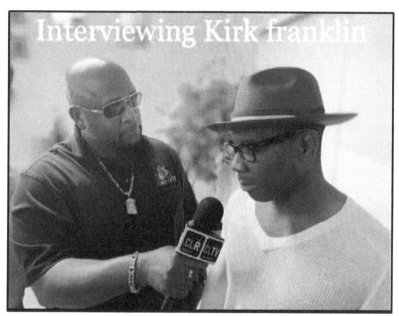

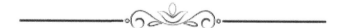
Interview with Kirk Franklin

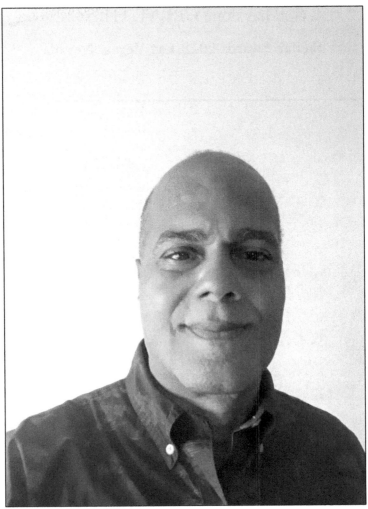

Michael Davis a.k.a Mike D. My business partner and mentor in the business. Thank you man for taking a young brown boy under your wings and letting me grow.

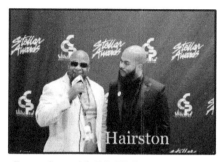

Interview with J.J. Hairston

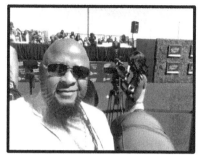

On the red carpet as Host
"Positive TV" Official Media.

I am so encouraged to share this journey also in pictures to help you envision your dream becoming a reality. No matter what's going on, don't stop believing and never surrender.

Everything is front of YOU!

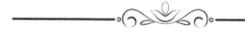

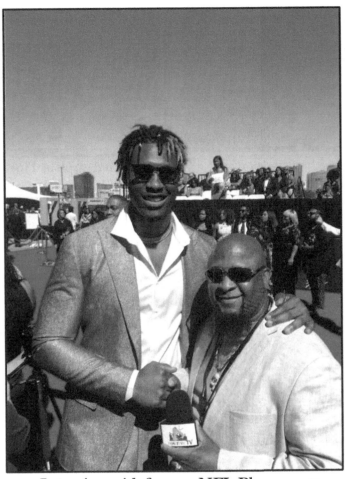

Interview with former NFL Player now
(Gospel) Radio Host

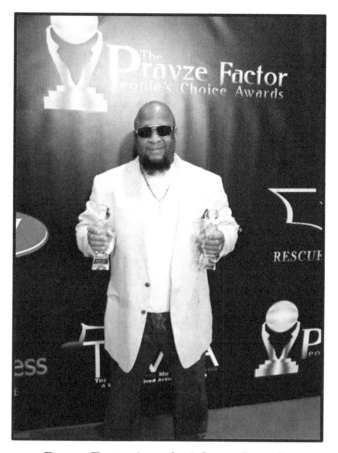

Prayze Factor Awards, Atlanta, Georgia

2015 [Winner of 2 awards]
TV Show and TV Host of the Year!

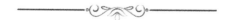

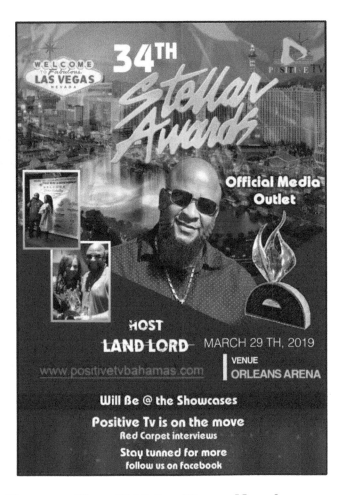

Showcase Host 2019 Las Vegas, Nevada
Stellar Awards Weekend

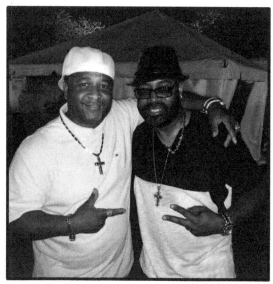

Hanging with J. Moss (Pastor and Recording Artist).
2nd concert –Nassau, Bahamas
Sponsored by the Ministry of Tourism.

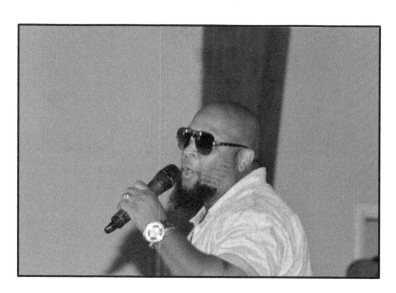

Stellar Awards 2019

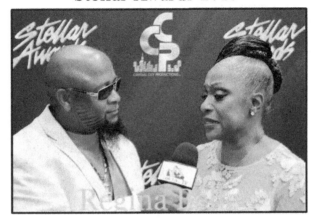

Interview with Regina Belle

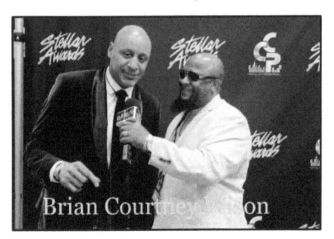

Interview with Brian Courtney Wilson
Interview with Cheryl Fortune
(Gospel Recording Artist)

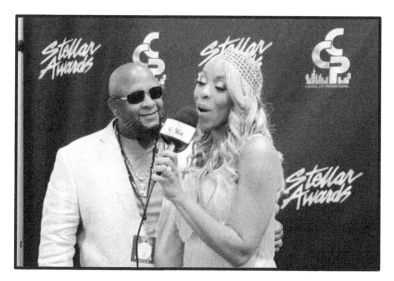

Interview with Gospel Recording Artist

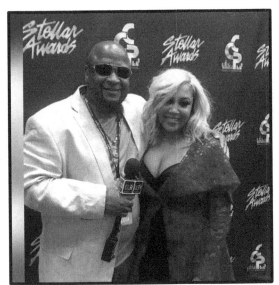

Interview with Cheryl Fortune,
Gospel Recording Artist

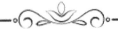

My *Mentor*, Dr. Myles Munroe

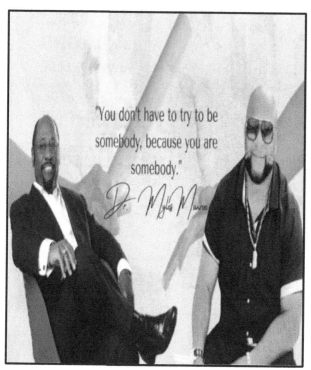

"You don't have to try to be somebody, because you are somebody."
Dr. Myles Munroe

Another wonderful moment. Blessed!

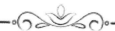

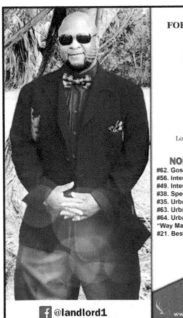

FOR YOUR CONSIDERATION
PLEASE *VOTE* FOR

LANDLORD

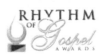

RHYTHM
OF *Gospel*
A W A R D S

July 20th, 2019 at 5:00 PM
Louisiana State University Auditorium
Baton Rouge, Louisiana

NOMINATION CATEGORIES:

#62. Gospel TV/Radio Show Of The Year
#56. Internet Radio Announcer Of The Year
#49. Internet Radio/Media Outlet Of The Year
#38. Special Event/Instrumental Artist Of The Year
#35. Urban Contemporary Male Vocalist
#63. Urban Contemporary Artist Of The Year
#64. Urban Contemporary Song Of The Year -
"Way Maker"
#21. Best Performance By Male Vocalist

UNLIMITED VOTING
please vote here

November 5th - March 1st
www.TheRhythmOfGospelAwards.com

@landlord1

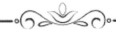

It speaks volumes... Praise God!

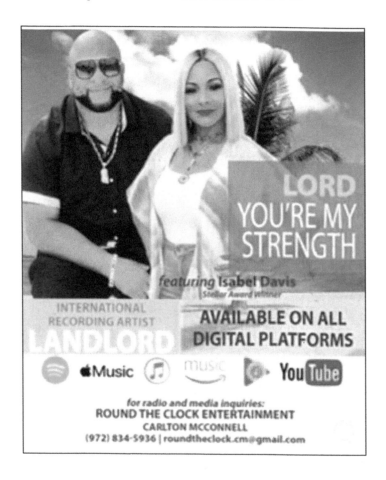

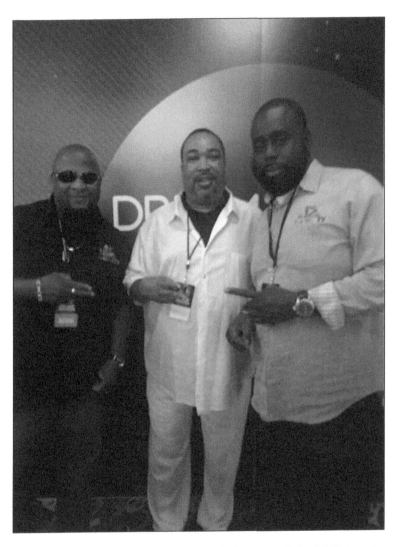

Left to right: Landlord, Carlton McConnell (middle) and Clifford Riley (end).

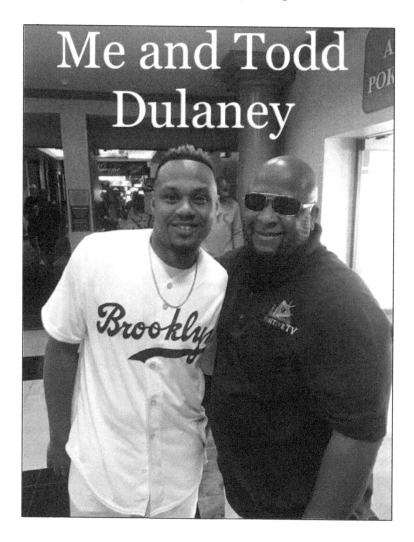

It Keeps Getting Better ... Thank YOU!

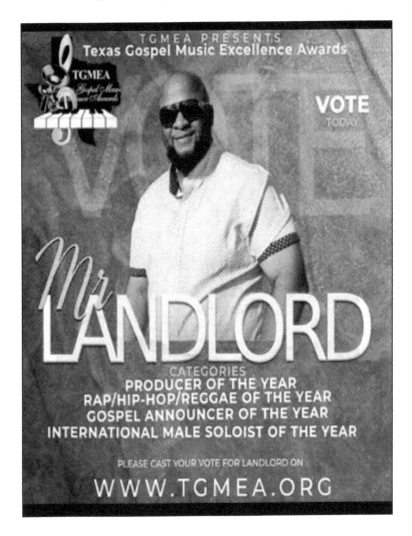

What an Amazing Journey!

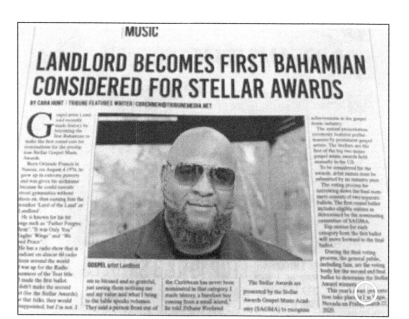

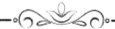

Siblings...We made it through!

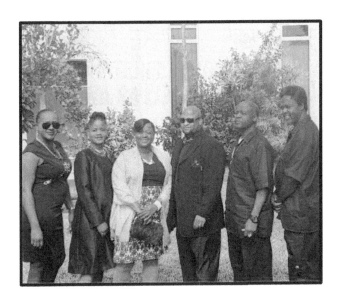

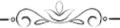

My Heart – My Jewel – My Mom

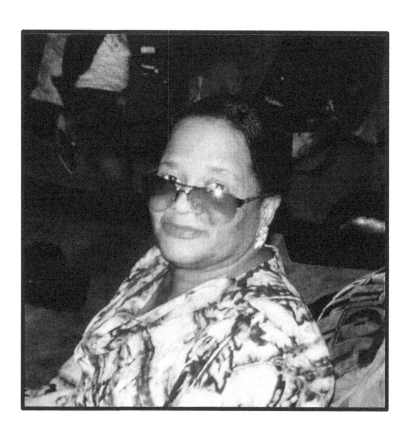

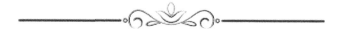

Proud Dad!!

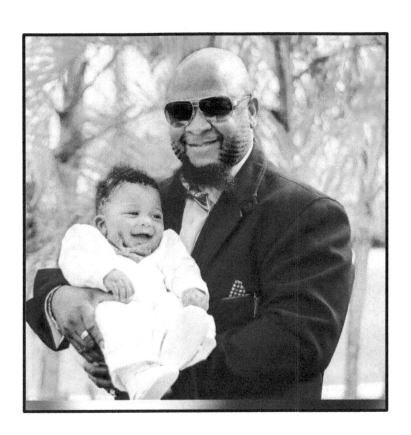

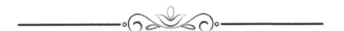

Meet the Family!

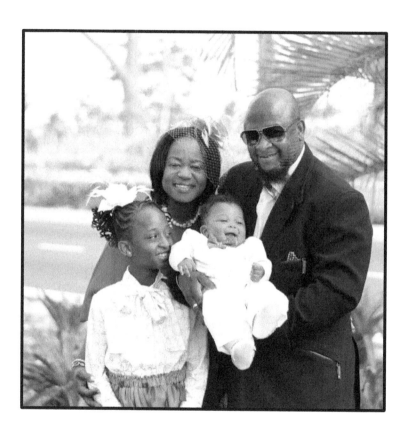

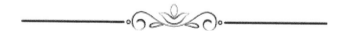

I didn't want this book to be an ordinary book about singing or traveling around the world, but I really desire to touch hearts and inspire God's people to trust Him.

In the worst case scenario when the adversary is beating you down, warring against your mind and emotions, I want to declare over your life: God will not leave you there if you simply look up and start trusting for a favorable outcome.

We're on this journey together and collectively we will win.

Thank you for supporting this project.

Contact Information

Phone: 242-4565596 954-9154117 (Global)
Email: Positivetvbahamas@gmail.com

Website: www.positivetvglobal.com

Facebook: Landlord242

Look forward to hearing from you!

Made in the USA
Columbia, SC
24 May 2022

60818725R00055